Endorse

"Prepare to Amaze yourself with the staying power you will gain from hypnosis to maintain your goals. You will provide your body with healthy foods and have the commitment to stay in motion. Jane Percy provides the tools you will need to make healthy choices and then engages your subconscious to make these changes seemingly effortlessly. Her soothing voice will provide complete relaxation as you change your thinking about foods and truly meet your goals to have a healthy and satisfied body and soul. You don't want to miss this opportunity to experience this book."

Dr. Caryn Nesbitt, Director Women's Care Center, Groton, CT

"Jane has pitched the message perfectly with a blend of encouragement and optimism underpinned by practical guidance and sound medical science. Even a skeptic and a hardened recidivist will be heartened by her book. Thanks for letting me review the document. It is an easy and plausible read even for a nay sayer like myself! Your style is just right, optimistic without being polyanna-ish. I found the text quite compelling."

Dr. Declan Doogan, SR. V.P., Pfizer. Inc.

"Jane Percy is a gifted hypnotherapist who supports her clients through the difficult and challenging process of re-learning how to eat properly for healthy and long-lasting weight loss."

Dr. Peter D'Adamo, author of
EAT RIGHT 4 YOUR BLOOD TYPE books.

Lighten Up!
Win at Losing

A Dynamic Program to Lose Weight and Gain Health Now

Jane H. Percy

New York

Lighten Up
Win At Losing: A dynamic program to lose weight and gain health now

ISBN 978-1-60037-773-0

Library of Congress Control Number: 2010925091

Morgan James Publishing
1225 Franklin Ave., STE 325
Garden City, NY 11530-1693
Toll Free 800-485-4943
www.MorganJamesPublishing.com

In an effort to support local communities, raise awareness and funds, Morgan James Publishing donates one percent of all book sales for the life of each book to Habitat for Humanity. Get involved today, visit **www.HelpHabitatForHumanity.org.**

Dedication

LIGHTEN UP! WIN AT LOSING is dedicated to all hardworking earth-keepers who raise delicious, organic, hormone-free food for our tables and who replenish the earth, not with chemicals, but with organic matter. Thank you for being good stewards and for feeding us well. I salute every farmer's market and every whole food store. It is also dedicated to fearless fishermen and women who bring fresh fish to us and who care about balanced harvesting of the sea, not exploitation. It is dedicated all who till the soil, whether it be a backyard garden or containers on your deck. From me and my family to you and yours … in very good health!

Acknowledgements

LIGHTEN UP! WIN AT LOSING grew out of my experiences as a medical hypnotherapist and the many opportunities I've had teaching food sense and weight health. And, of course, there were many helpers along the way:

Thanks to Evie and Bill, my parents, whose shared interest in gardens and home grown vegetables influenced my appreciation of organically grown food. My father who is now in his ninth decade still plants his garden every spring and he encourages other seniors in his community to join in.

Amy Dunion; a leader in William H. Backus Hospital's holistic health community and Lynn McCarthy of the Lawrence & Memorial Hospital Wellness Center orchestrated my classes. Bless you both.

The late Dr. Caryn Nesbitt both inspired and supported me and my writing. Caryn was eloquent in all things and she is sorely missed.

Dr. Declan Doogan, Fellow of the Royal College of Physicians of Glasgow and President of Research and Development, Amarin Company, reviewed my manuscript with great care. Thank you Dec and Dorothy for your friendship and encouragement.

I'm ever grateful to writers Gracelyn Guyol and Ruth Crocker for their editing expertise and friendship.

Thank you, Joan Farley! Your enthusiasm and energy fueled the success of our *Lighten Up* Programs. Our wonderful and talented designer, Marie Carija, fostered the shape and form of this book.

I'm grateful to my agent, Bob Silverstein and all the gang at Morgan James Publishing. Thank you Richard Sutphen for introducing me to Bob Silverstein.

And finally, three cheers to all my *Lighten Up* students. Keep up the good work; the world needs you to be fit and feisty.

Contents

Affirmation:
"I eat less, exercise more, and enjoy healthy changes in my body and my life."

1.   Not a Diet, But a Way of Life

We are the most overfed, over-medicated and under-nourished population in the world. Our children are becoming fatter and unhealthier by the moment. Weight related illnesses threaten to overwhelm our already overburdened health care system. Why is it that the wealthiest nation in the world has such an unhealthy population? What can you do to get slender and stay that way? This book with CD gives you a pleasant, sensible, sustain-

> When healthy thoughts and choices become healthy actions, wonderful things happen.

able way of getting to a healthy weight. Think of it as your very own slimming kit. Living Lightly is the way to health and longevity. Once you master the simple principles of this program, you'll never have to diet again. For the last eight years, I've been teaching *Lighten Up, Win At Losing*, a dynamic weight loss program that combines hypnosis with an eating concept I call *Positive Eating*…not a diet, but a way of life. *The Lighten Up* way is a very effective way to achieve and maintain a healthy weight, and create longevity and wellbeing. A lifelong interest in food, exercise, and optimal health combined with my passionate interest in the mind—along with the power of hypnosis to help you change your mind—impels me to share this information with you.

I've taught *Lighten Up* methods to hundreds of people of all ages and walks of life. During that time, my students have taught me as well. I've learned from them that old habits of unhealthy overeating can transform into new health patterns when the mind and the body are in agreement. When healthy thoughts and choices become healthy actions, wonderful things happen.

The *Lighten Up* way is not a diet in the usual sense. Most people in my classes are experts on dieting, reminiscent of Mark Twain who famously quipped that quitting smoking was easy, he'd done it hundreds of times!

Change your mind about food and you'll change your whole life. Stop dieting now and begin to truly understand food. All of us, especially our children, need to become lean and strong again. This begins by changing our value system, moving from eating highly processed foods, from using food as emotional comfort, from failing to use our bodies as they were designed—which is to be in motion.

Did you learn to use food as consolation, reward, comfort? Did someone give you a cookie to distract you during a moment of childhood upset or as a reward? If so, you may have gotten stuck in the belief that food is comfort, love, or reward. You can shift your thinking. The main difference between overweight people and people who maintain fit, slender bodies is that slim people think of food as fuel; they make discerning choices about

> Change your mind about food, change your whole life. Stop dieting. Begin to truly understand food.

what constitutes fuel and what does not. As you read *Lighten Up, Win at Losing* and begin to practice hypnotic re-learning, you'll be able to shift from the old and damaging way you thought about food to a new empowering view. Food is fuel! You and your wonderful body deserve to have high quality fuel to energize and renew your being. And yes, there can be enormous pleasure and enjoyment in eating this way.

Affirmation:
"I am doing well and I enjoy turning old cravings into healthy actions."

2. Hypnosis Gets Me Started, Helps Me Lose, and Keeps Me Going

Hypnosis is a pleasant and relaxing way of breaking old, unhealthy patterns of overeating, under nourishing, and yo-yo dieting. Hypnosis helps free you of old habits, cravings, and binge eating; it can literally help you *change your mind* about food once and for all. It also helps you jump-start your healthy exercise program and stick with it. You have already been hypnotized by television ads to believe that food IS emotional nourishment. Remember "Nothing says lovin' like somethin' from the oven" or "Bake Someone Happy." Your computer screen and your TV are highly hypnotic.

> Research shows that dieters lose twice as much weight when hypnosis is combined with healthy food and exercise and they keep the weight off longer.

Therapeutic Hypnosis negotiates agreement between mind AND body (this is *real* will power) so that change occurs, and more importantly, so that change is sustainable and life-long. Research shows that dieters lose twice as much weight when hypnosis is combined with healthy food and exercise and they keep the weight off longer.[1]

So, this little kit has what you need to get started on the rest of your life as a healthy, confident consumer of food. By listening to the your hypnosis sound track (you will find download instructions in the resources section of the book, chapter 22), you'll discover that when you change your mind about food, your body will naturally adjust its weight downward. When you add a little consistent exercise, your strong and slender body will emerge. Believe me, it's in there!

Your thinking mind does everything it can to resist change and it doesn't govern will power. Perhaps this is why just when you decide that today is the day to start losing weight, you hear a little voice inside that says "Aw come on, just one more brownie or ice cream cone...you deserve it" and the next moment you make an unhealthy choice and feel guilty about it. Your subconscious mind (the mind you activate in hypnosis) is in charge of will power. It is about 8 to 10 times stronger than your thinking mind. Let your sub-conscious mind help you carry out your desire to change your mind

---

1   Journal of Consulting and Clinical Psychology, 64 (3), 517-
   519..Hypnotic Enhancement of Cognitive Behavior Weight
   Loss Treatments- Another Meta-Reanalysis. Irving Kirsch,
   University of CT, 1996.

about food, and exercise as you become lean, mean, and delicious. You'll fine it easier and easier to pass up foods that trigger weight gain, making healthier choices.

You'll want to listen to the *Lighten Up* hypnosis recording once a day in a quiet place (not while driving or operating machinery) where you won't be interrupted. The recording is 24 minutes long. It will help activate your will power reserves through your imagination—for this is the place where change begins: in the subconscious mind. There are other wonderful health benefits that come from listening. When you listen consistently, your blood pressure, mood, and energy levels will improve almost immediately. We know that stress is more fattening than any food you can eat, so the quality of relaxation achieved when you listen will help your body regulate its weight downward. In other words, hypnotic relaxation is great for your metabolism but it does more than that to assist your body.

Your sub-conscious mind (the mind you activate in hypnosis) is in charge of will power. It is about 8 to 10 times stronger than your thinking mind. Let your sub-conscious mind help you carry out your desire to change your mind about food and exercise as you become lean, mean, and delicious. You'll find it easier and easier to pass up foods that trigger weight gain, making healthier choices.

Hypnosis effectively lowers cortisol, blood pressure, blood sugar, and cholesterol. The images and sounds in the recording are truly medicine, but without any negative side effects, offering you a reduction in your weight and stress levels. Hypnosis is truly mind and body medicine.

Many people in my classes comment on better quality sleep, a reduction in painful joints, stiff limbs, and improved focus and mental endurance. All talk about how regular listening helps them to feel more relaxed, more in control. They learn to listen daily and to supplement listening by practicing self-hypnosis which is covered in chapter 19.

People sometimes ask me: "When is the best time for me to listen?" My answer is to listen at different times and see when you feel you get the most out of it. If you constantly fall asleep, say, in the evening, try another time to listen. However, the best time to listen is when you CAN listen, because the important thing is to listen once a day, every day.

At the end of the hypnosis segment there will be an opportunity to learn and practice self-hypnosis. You'll be able to hypnotize yourself in less time than it takes to wash your hands, staying focused and committed to healthy goals. What a wonderful and powerful tool this is for converting cravings into healthy actions. Self-hypnosis is like sending a Text Message to yourself to exercise today, to eat a little less and focus on intensely nutrient-rich foods, saying no to foods that aren't really food; just empty calories that cause inflammation, disease and excess body weight.

There are many ways that hypnosis heals long term, subconscious weight and food issues. I recently worked with Joan, an attractive, vivacious woman in her mid-forties. She felt overwhelmed by her inability to attain and maintain her ideal weight and after many diet failures she came to see me. She had recently been through an intense period of stress and the painful loss of both parents. She also seemed to have many non-specific worries and fears; she was anxious a good deal of the time. We had good results in reducing her stress levels by increasing her daily exercise, adjusting her food choices and utilizing hypnosis to create focus and calm. Still, there was something standing in the way of her weight loss success.

So, I guided her back in time hypnotically (this is called hypnotic regression) and gave her the suggestion that she would be able to easily drift back in time to a significant memory that would illuminate her current situation. She remembered, during the summer before her 7th grade year, wearing a pair of shorts that no longer fit her... they were last years shorts and just too tight. I asked her if there was anything else that "didn't fit" and she immediately connected to the intensely uncomfortable memory of moving that same fall to a new school and all the self-conscious teen triggers were in full force. She felt anxious, uncomfortable and fearful about fitting in. At that point I called on a "Wise Guide" to help her see things in another light. The voice of inner wisdom said: "Your weight was healthy. You just outgrew your shorts and that is normal for a 13 year old girl. Your body was changing and it was time for a new pair of shorts." Still there was more…the theme of things not "fitting" and feeling a loss of control had more to reveal.

While still in hypnosis, I moved Joan forward in time to a significant adult memory. She remembered after the birth of her second child that her doctor told her she was fat. Her weight, a few months after childbirth, was actually normal but she believed her doctor. Once again, her Wise Guide was called upon and spoke to her doctor and told him that his remark was hurtful. Her Body Mass Index was a normal 23 and so her Wise Guide informed the doctor that he was incorrect and Joan was able to feel more in control.

Before emerging Joan from hypnosis, we spent some time integrating these two memories. It was clear that when things "didn't fit" or felt out of control, Joan had a tendency to focus inordinately on her weight just as she did that summer before 7th grade.

Also, she tended to give authority to others rather than trusting her inner guidance. She emerged from that session with a greater sense of peace and self-trust with readiness to accomplish her healthy weight goals.

The subconscious mind is a vast library of memory. This memory bank retains beliefs, feelings and stories that influence every aspect of our lives and every choice we make.

Here's another example of the power of the subconscious mind: Pat, age 60, was beautiful and charismatic. Everyone in her Lighten Up class enjoyed being with her. She was also diabetic and extremely overweight as were many in her family. When given the instruction to go back in time to a significant memory (in hypnosis), Pat remembered her older brother (she was 6) telling her over and over and in a taunting way that she was fat. And she said aloud "You think this is fat? I'll show you fat." Each successive year, Pat gained more and more ("I'll show you!") and her adult life was fraught with serious health conditions. With a little hypnotic prompting, her Wise Guide asked her if she could forgive her brother and let go of this argument or challenge which had controlled her entire life. During this emotional but healing inner conversation, Pat was able to commit to a healthier path to finally release the need to prove something, even if to her detriment, to her brother.

IMAGINE

You are surrounded by waves of peace, comfort and calm. In this place of serenity, the voice of your Wise Guide or inner wisdom is clearly audible to you. In the presence of your own wisdom, you find your deepest truth. It is as though you've always known what you need to do to thrive....and so you do.

Affirmation:
"I choose high value foods, eat less, and feel satisfied and nourished."

3. Healthy Habits For Life

The following suggestions may surprise you. Please give them a try and see what a difference they make.

Replace Fluid

When you awaken, replace fluid lost during sleep by drinking 16 oz. of pure, fresh water. Do this every day and you will notice how it improves your complexion and your mood. It also helps to awaken metabolic capability.

Eat breakfast!

This is the most important meal of the day. I'm afraid for many of us it is either skipped or consists of coffee and something sugary... sorry Dunkin Donuts, this little book is not going to improve your sales. Skipping breakfast literally disables your metabolism, your body's precious ability to utilize food as nourishment without

> Eat a good breakfast and turn your metabolic switch to the ON position for the day.

storing it as excess fat. Eat a good breakfast and turn your metabolic switch to the ON position for the day.

Good things for breakfast

Eggs…don't cook the yolk all the way (soft boil, poach or easy over and easy on the oil). Why? Eggs are a perfect food and the egg's cholesterol content is balanced by the lecithin it contains which is a natural emulsifier (fat buster). However, lecithin is destroyed when the egg yolk is overcooked. I'll tell you later on how white potatoes are hurting us and making us fat, so please, no home fries with your egg. How about some lean turkey bacon for extra crunch and additional morning protein to energize your whole day?

Enjoy and amplify the nutritional content of this first meal of your day with fresh fruit (not juice, it is too sugary), sprouted grain products (see list in back of book) with pure, natural peanut, walnut, or almond butter. Please don't eat peanut butter that has added sugar and hydrogenated fat (lethal). Get the good stuff. Enjoy low fat yogurt, protein shakes, whole oats oatmeal (not the tasteless, over sweetened packaged instant variety).

My favorite breakfast memory of all time was one spring when I was given freshly caught wild trout and strawberries by my New Hampshire host. This was many years ago but I remember it still…a perfect combination of lean protein, freshly picked fruit and the taste of a nearby river with sun blessed berries. Getting good quality protein into this first, all important meal of the day will help your body remain energized AND it will help you lose weight because your metabolic light switch is now turned ON! Be creative and know that most of the "bready" things we tend to eat for breakfast are overly refined. English muffins, bagels, white bread, God forbid, frozen waffles, pancakes—yikes, the calories go….right to your waistline. These poor quality carbohydrates sap your energy by raising blood sugar at a rapid rate. By mid-morning you'll be dragging and craving more of the same.

Start your day with high value protein and watch your waistline get smaller and smaller and your energy soar!

Coffee Break

Why is it that when we have coffee, we add sweet things (coffee cake!!)? In the middle of the morning I would encourage you to have a big glass of water and see if you really need anything more. If so, have an apple or a few nuts. People who are most successful at losing weight find it helpful to eat well at mealtime and avoid in between meal snacks. You'll have to find your way with this. Your me-

> Foods with healthy fat and fiber (nuts, for instance) will hold hunger at bay and keep blood sugar stable.

tabolism likes it best when you allow at least four hours between breakfast and lunch. If you stay well hydrated, and if you've eaten a good balance of protein, fat, fiber (those wonderful nut butters or a handful of nuts), and slow carbohydrates★ you won't be ravenous. If you have hypoglycemia, snacking thoughtfully will help to maintain blood sugar. Some mid-morning suggestions: nut butter or hummus on rice crackers or celery, low-fat yogurt. Foods with healthy fat and fiber (nuts, for instance) will hold hunger at bay and keep blood sugar stable. Sugary carbohydrates stimulate the worst responses in your body especially converting food to stored fat instead of energy. Your morning donut sets you up for day long sugar cravings.

Lunch
Once again, steer clear of bready foods (grinders, sandwiches, pizza). Instead, enjoy fresh soups (the non-creamy types with broth and lots of fresh vegetables and some protein), and salads with protein, lots of variety and crunch. Croutons add calories so experiment with slivered almonds, walnuts or pumpkin seeds for crunch. Please do enjoy full fat olive oil on your salads. Creamy dressings and diet dressings will make it harder for you to lose weight but real olive oil with a bit of vinegar or lemon will help you lose. Olive oil in small amounts is your weight-busting friend for it is a slimming, heart-healthy fat.

★ Slow carbs are those which are high in fiber and low on the glycemic index. You'll find more about these beneficial carbohydrates on page eighteen.

Snacks

If dinner is more than five hours later than lunch, you'll need a carefully planned snack to stay energized and focused—and to keep hunger from becoming too fierce. A crisp apple is a great portable choice. Celery with nut butter, a few rice crackers with hummus or a little goat cheese, walnuts or almonds…good choices for the late afternoon. Have some green tea and BREATHE…four really deep breaths will lower your blood pressure while bumping your metabolism up a notch. The accumulation of stress often results in excessive eating, snacking, and calorie overload at the end of the day. This may be the perfect time to take a walk or to listen to your hypnosis recording.

Energy Bars Aren't

A word about energy/protein bars and sports drinks: they are highly processed and loaded with sugar and additives. Please switch to real food. There was a woman in one of my Lighten Up classes who insisted that her brand of protein bar made a great breakfast. When she brought it to class I asked her to read the ingredients aloud…it went something like this: soy, corn syrup (death by sugar), whey powder (dairy) and chocolate… also it was very caloric at 300 calories per bar, but had very little nutrition (fuel). A better choice would be a slice of Manna or gluten free rice almond bread with a tablespoon of walnut butter which provides fuel in the form of: fiber (8 grams), protein (10), beneficial fat (the slenderizing kind), and slow carbohydrates. You can make one of these sandwiches in about 40 seconds and they keep well in a baggie for a couple of days. These wholesome snacks are delicious and convenient as well as inexpensive. They are fuel-filled while free of additives and preservatives. Add an apple to this mini-sandwich for a wholesome hearty snack or a meal substitute. By the way, this is how I survive airplane food! Please say no to energy and protein bars and yes to snacks that truly DO energize you without elevating your blood sugar and activating cravings.

Sports drinks
Sports drinks are potassium enriched liquid candy. They have way too much sugar to be beneficial. If you took a Gatorade drink and combined 1 part drink to 3 parts sparkling water you'd have a refreshing drink, but drinking these sugary drinks at full strength is not beneficial. A marathoner can metabolize all the sugar from such a drink but most of us haven't just run 26 miles. For thirst, and to keep your mineral intake balanced, enjoy fresh water with a handful of grapes. You'll get all the health benefits you need without any of the toxic additives or sugar that's found in most sports drinks.

Slow carbohydrates
Slow carbohydrates are the ones you want to eat: legumes, brown rice and whole grains, fruit, and vegetables (leave the skin on for added fiber and nutrients) because they

help you maintain a steady blood sugar. Fast carbohydrates are baked goods and deserts, commercial pasta, white potatoes, and sugary drinks and candy. These raise your blood sugar which leads to insulin resistance, diabetes, metabolic syndrome and excess weight. Always choose slow carbs…they are your weight management allies.

> Slow carbohydrates are the ones you want to eat: legumes, brown rice and whole grains, fruit, and vegetables because they help you maintain a steady blood sugar.

Energy Bars and sports drinks are the result of convenience driven consumerism – a very successful marketing campaign to get you to buy and consume drinks and snacks that impact your weight and health. If you read labels on these items closely, you'll see that they don't contain much food or fuel. Shop for more natural convenience foods (unsalted nuts, fruit, wheat-free crackers, Manna bread). It's your life and your body and you deserve it.

Dinner

Dinner is ideally a smaller, lighter meal than lunch because your body can't metabolize a heavy meal at the end of the day. Just think how many people eat steak, potatoes, and bread at the end of the day. Add cheesecake (yikes!) or ice cream and your inflammation driven weight gain mechanism is engaged. No wonder nearly everyone is on statin drugs. Your hard working liver objects to this food insult by producing excess cholesterol and generating other inflammatory responses. Fish is always a good food choice in the evening along with a fresh salad and a steamed vegetable. In Lighten Up classes I encourage people to stop eating potatoes except for sweet potatoes—a superior food.

Potatoes ... Do We Need Them?

About potatoes: A baked one is decent food especially if you enjoy the skin, which is where most of the fiber and vitamins are. A dollop of low fat yogurt on half a baked potato (with skin for fiber and vital nutrients) is very satisfying. Our ghastly restaurant habit of piling food on top of a mound of mashed potatoes is making us a sick, overweight nation; add some white bread and the spiral downward is well underway. Your bathroom scale knows this all too well! Forget French fries...ok, I might have three a year, but they are not a valuable food EVER. Remember this: fast food and junk food are NOT food... not for a lean, mean, gorgeous you. If you crave the crunch of fries, try sweet potato fries that you bake until crisp; they are a healthy alternative.

Pasta

About pasta: we eat too much of it and many of the sauces are fatty. In Italy, pasta is served as a very small part of the meal; here in the US it tends to be the whole meal. I like the wheat-free pastas. I encourage my *Lighten Up* students to eat those sparingly with toppings that have fresh vegetables, protein (seafood, lean meat, or tofu), and delightful, fresh herbs with a bit of olive oil and garlic. If you are eating pasta, make salad your main course and pasta the side order. If you get the ratios right, you'll be able to enjoy many favorite foods without hurting yourself or your midriff.

Dining Out

If you tend to dine out a lot, enjoy places that prepare fresh fish really well and know that adding a salad and a vegetable makes a great meal. Remember, too, that YOU are the customer and that meat topped with cheese or a rich sauce isn't going to help your waistline. Please give yourself permission to ask for adaptations so that the meal you receive is the one you want and need. When you get in the habit of ordering fuel instead of food, you'll know that you are on the path to slender health.

I enjoy some of our neighborhood restaurants in Mystic and Stonington and I talk to waiters and owners a lot. These hard working people really do want you to have the meal you need and desire so it is your absolute right to ask for menu adaptations and substitutions. It it OK to leave the unhealthy toppings and sides in the kitchen—all you need to do is ask.

Don't let guilt or anyone bully you into eating something that doesn't nourish you or to eat more than your body knows it needs.

Portions

Never eat everything! Did you grow up believing that cleaning your plate was a good habit? Many of us did. Perhaps like mine, your parents remembered Depression days when food was scarce. The pendulum has swung in the opposite direction. Now, we are sick from overeating. You are a grown up…you can decide how much food is enough. Don't let guilt or anyone bully you into eating something that doesn't nourish you. Don't eat more than your body knows it needs. Most entrees are twice the size you need so plan on eating half and taking the rest home. You can make sensible food choices and you don't need anyone's permission. Hooray!

The Two Cup Rule

Restaurant size dinner plates are just getting bigger and bigger. And the dinner plates we use at home are also very, very large. If you switch to luncheon size plates (8") you'll find it easier to adjust your meal portions, thus comfortably eating less each day. As Dr. Barry Sears points out in his *Zone Diet* book, to get to a healthy nutritional balance, divide your plate the following way: protein (lean meat or fish) 4 oz. or about the size of the palm of your hand, vegetable (one cup), and salad (about 2 cups). You'll see, there's no room for mashed potatoes, French fries or pasta. You could add a small amount of winter squash, sweet potato or unrefined brown rice. Your stomach is designed to comfortably manage about 2 to 2 ½ cups of food per meal. If you cup your hands together, the capacity you create is about 2 cups so you always have a measuring system with you. If you select high value foods and eat moderate portions slowly, you will be satisfied.

Social Choices

One *Lighten Up* student, a successful professional woman, and mother of three, spoke tearfully about a family gathering. She was scolded for saying a polite "no thank you" to her mother's killer (really) potato salad. Family patterns around food are either healthy or tyrannously unhealthy. Take a little time to evaluate your family pattern and give yourself a *Get Out Of Jail* card NOW! You can and should love 'em all, but you don't have to inherit unhealthy food behaviors which become part of family culture. Now is the time to be liberated, to Lighten Up! Do you have friends who only want to be with you at the pizza parlor or the buffet? Our food habits often affect our social choices and vice versa.

Eat Slowly

When you eat slowly, savoring each flavor while chewing at a deliberately more relaxed rate, you give your body time to register signals of near fullness. It takes about twenty minutes for this complex series of signals to register in both the brain and stomach. If you gulp or rush through your meal, you will likely overeat from bypassing these helpful signals of fullness. Rushing through meals makes us fat as well as seriously impacting our digestive process.

Small Meals with Variety

Small meals that have variety in textures and tastes satisfy more than a large quantity of one food. If you eat mostly processed food, your appetite for flavor variety is less likely to be satisfied so you'll eat more and weigh more. The larger the range of flavors in your meals—savory, tart, bitter, tangy, spicy—the less food you'll need to feel satisfied.

It is time to change our value system around food. Eating everything is not healthy. Eating slowly, mindfully and stopping before you become full is a healthy way to aid digestion and weight. Eating less but selecting high value, nutrient rich whole food is NOURISHMENT.

Don't Drink While You Eat

This may surprise you, but the habit of drinking beverages with our meals actually is most unhealthy. Drink lots of water, green tea, sparkling water all day long but don't drink anything with your meal. Why? Adding liquids while you eat inhibits your natural, most necessary and beneficial production of saliva, the first, and most essential step in the digestive process. Also, when you chew food thoroughly and salivate properly, you are less likely to have digestive upsets AND you often feel more satisfied, tending to eat less. The water you gulp during mealtime shuts down your salivary production, actually diluting the stomach acid NEEDED for proper digestion. Your pets already know this...watch them eat and notice that they don't go from their food bowl to their water bowl and back. When they eat, they chew and salivate; water intake is separate. Make this simple change and notice that your digestion is much more efficient and comfortable. This new habit will reduce acid reflux, acid indigestion and GERD. Less food will satisfy you.

Heartburn

Eating the wrong foods at the wrong time and in unhealthy quantities is creating another health concern. A recent *Journal of the American Medical Association* reveals that heart-burn drugs are linked to increased likelihood of hip and bone fracture, often leading to life threatening conditions. If you have heartburn, you'll improve rapidly by following these common sense eating habits: eating slowly, chewing thoroughly, not drinking liquids with your food, choosing high value (unprocessed) food.

her favorite exercise was to sit and read. I'm sure she was doing the best she could but you don't have to be a dietician to see how her eating and sedentary habits were making her sick and likely depressed.

My mother

She grew up eating the way her mother did. I was one of five children, so I imagine feeding all of us was a miracle. In my early childhood, I remember a lot of creamed tuna on toast and summer meals of hamburgers and platters of both farm fresh corn on the cob and sliced garden tomatoes with mayo. Somewhere in her forties, recurring heart disease began to trouble her. Then one day my mother read Adelle Davis's wonderful book *Eat Right To Keep Fit* and a food revolution in our family began. She bought a super-duper juicer and truly worked hard at bringing healthier food to our table.

In addition to chasing five children, she took up walking, golf and tennis; overcoming her family's sedentary pattern. The point of all this is to say that you can overcome your family history around food and exercise. Your biography doesn't have to be your biology. You are what you eat, what you think, what you feel. You are what you believe. Your body and all of its miraculous cells reflect every belief you have about yourself. Are you ready to develop Positive Eating habits?

I hope you'll take a moment to reflect on your family experiences; especially learned or observed habits. This is a good starting place to create new ideals and values about food and exercise.

One very successful *Lighten Up* student remembered, while in hypnosis, that her mother constantly commented on how skinny she was by saying: "Don't worry, you'll fill out" and years later in her 50s she began to fill out and then become very, very overweight. Through a dialogue process with her mother's memory, she was able to release all sub-conscious need to "fill out" so she could emerge from hypnosis and succeed at losing weight.

What are the stated and unstated food habits and beliefs in your family that adversely affect your weight? Are you ready to identify and release them for the sake of your health and well being? As you become more and more consciously aware, you'll be able to make gradual changes while you continue to detach yourself from unhelpful family food habits.

Remember that food is such a central part of family culture; whatever you learn from your family will continue to influence you, positively or adversely, until you "change your mind" and establish habits and choices that are best for you. Don't worry, you won't be excommunicated if you say "no thank you" to Aunt Mary's cheesecake. Just hug her instead and then say "no thank you."

IMAGINE

Picture yourself enjoying a peaceful, healthful, balanced meal with family or friends. You are having a delightful time, eating mindfully and moderately...you are feeling very comfortable. The pleasurable sensations of taste combine beautifully with conversation... and so this meal is a sacred blessing.

Affirmation:
"I listen closely and deeply to the messages and needs of my body and nourish it thoughtfully."

5.   Blood Type and pH

Blood Type

A mainstay in my *Lighten Up* classes are Dr. Peter D'Adamo's wonderful books on *Eat Right 4 Your Type*. Do you know your blood type? A generation ago, blood type was considered general knowledge; your family physician probably had your type on record. If you've donated blood, your Red Cross donor's card will have your blood type on it. Or, you can use a home blood typing kit which takes about three minutes.

I recommend reading *Eat Right 4 Your Blood Type* and following the food guidelines therein. I've used this information in all of my Lighten Up classes and it has helped hundreds of people lose weight and recover from high cholesterol, high blood pressure, arthritis pain, and digestive complaints. One *Lighten Up* student (a gentleman in his 50s) found that once he began to make healthy blood type choices, he lost weight and no longer needed his eye glasses. Your immune system will love you for eating this new way and you'll find that many chronic complaints resolve.

pH

Another excellent approach to weight, wellness, and longevity is to be aware of your body's pH balance. An acid body is often stressed and overweight, subject to pain and dis-ease. An alkaline body is more able to maintain optimal weight and to defend itself against colds, flu, and life threatening diseases. I love Dr. Baroody's wonderful book *Alkalize or Die* (see Resources, chapter 21) and it will help you choose alkaline foods.

A body goes out of alkaline balance fairly easily but 20 minutes of hypnosis (your free recording) will actually help you restore this precious balance so that you can recover from highly acidic food, a toxic or stressful time in your life or from lack of sleep. Testing saliva and urine regularly will help you be aware of your body's subtle response to food. A healthy body easily maintains a pH of about 7.2.

Interestingly, hypnosis is very alkalizing. If you've had a stressful day compounded by eating an imbalance of acid producing foods (processed food, flabby carbs, too much meat), fifteen minutes of hypnotic relaxation will assist in returning to healthful alkaline balance which is necessary to achieve and maintain a healthy weight. It is also worthwhile to replace "acid" thoughts and words (criticism, judgments, disapproval) with toxin free thoughts and words (approval, tolerance, and acceptance).

IMAGINE

Take a moment to enjoy a deep, restorative breath. Let your eyes close as you picture a cool, lush, fragrant forest. You are surrounded by various shades of green and perhaps you notice the musical sound of a nearby waterfall or mountain stream. Feelings of stillness and peace move through you. All is well.

Affirmation:

"More and more I enjoy fresh, wholesome, colorful, energy giving food."

6.   Choices

Diet Food is awful for you. It isn't fuel! Eat real food… very fresh, unprocessed real food. Most of the food on the shelves in your grocery store and also in your kitchen cupboards has little or no real nourishment. **Highly processed food**, full of preservatives and additives will have a toxic effect on your body and you'll never feel fully satisfied eating it. **Food with a long shelf life** might be good for the food industry but I guarantee it has very little ener-

A good rule of thumb when you are shopping is to fill your basket with fresh vegetables (lots of color and variety) and fruit, a little lean protein, fresh organic eggs (to be enjoyed in moderation), whole grains and legumes.

getic life force to sustain you. A good rule of thumb when you are shopping is to fill your basket with fresh vegetables (lots of color and variety) and fruit, a little lean protein, fresh organic eggs (to be enjoyed in mod-

37

eration), whole grains and legumes. Stay away from the other isles—the outer perimeter of most grocery stores is where you'll find fuel. The other isles are designed to be very seductive…you know what I'm talking about, chips, baked goods etc. There's not much in the deli that's worthwhile either; maybe some real baked turkey or lean beef. Highly processed deli meats are salty with many toxic additives and these do affect your ability to burn stored fat and maintain alkaline balance.

Yes, you'll want to keep a supply of frozen vegetables and fruit in your freezer. I love ground turkey and turkey cutlets which also freeze well. If you haven't had time to shop, you can prepare a balanced meal that your body will utilize well and appreciate. Add a frozen vegetable, brown rice or half a baked sweet potato and you'll be able to prepare a meal even when you don't have a lot of fresh food around.

All artificial sweeteners are programmed to make you fat (they misinform and confuse your body's response to sweetness) and to make you crave them.

If you give up all diet beverages you'll be taking a big step—an important one for your health. These drinks are so addictive that I've had clients who have needed hypnosis to help them overcome their diet cola addiction.

Sodas have no value whatsoever and they are highly toxic to your body. Keep reading, for some delightful, healthy beverages, but you already know that **WATER**, pure, clean water is your weight loss ally. Your body is over seventy percent water and so its daily fluid requirements need to be met for you to thrive. Fresh water is a beauty elixir and a waistline trimmer. Often a drink of water will reduce hunger pangs and cravings. Make spicy ginger ale with soda water, grated fresh ginger, a squeeze of lemon juice and stevia to sweeten. You might like to add fresh squeezed lemon or lime to your water—this is very alkalizing.

Sparkling water with a splash of unsweetened cranberry, pomegranate, or grape juice is a great drink and a much better choice than soda every time.

By now you've heard that green tea has antioxidant benefits (oxidation is what makes apples and bananas turn brown when exposed to air...a kind of "rust" if you will). Green tea also has thermogenic benefits which means that it helps your metabolism (your fat burning mechanism, among other things). If you are brewing green tea you'll know it's the real thing if the wet tea leaves are really bright green. You might want to try other herbal teas for variety and wellbeing...please say no to all soda; it is just liquid candy.

In general, **fruit juice** is not a worthwhile food. Instead of orange juice (highly concentrated and sugary) enjoy a whole orange. Canned juices are too highly refined and sugary to be of any benefit. If you like fresh juice, consider getting a juicer and experiment with both low sugar fruit and green vegetable juices. These juices are packed with nutrients and life-giving enzymes and and they make wonderful in between meal snacks. Once you start eating live, unadulterated whole foods, your palate will change and you won't want anything else.

Sugar is on the *Lighten Up* hit list. We eat way too much of it. In the simplest terms, the more you eat the more you desire. The vicious sugar cycle is a major hurdle for many who want to lose weight. By adding naturally sweet food such as whole, fresh fruit to your diet and saying no thank you to dessert, you'll be able to break this cycle.

Of all the things in our national food supply, high fructose corn syrup is one of the most insidious and is highly contributory to our national obesity profiles. It is in everything and is even used to glaze hamburger buns before they are baked to make them look more appetizing and it makes your appetite go wild! Reading labels carefully will help to eliminate this syrup from your home. If you and your doctor are not happy with your cholesterol numbers or blood sugar, you'll certainly want to eliminate corn syrup completely from your diet.

An exercise we do in *Lighten Up* classes is to visualize sweetness in life...friends, family, pets and all the elements that help to create joy. There are also acts of unexpected kindness and generosity, moments of gratitude and feeling our deservedness.

By focusing on gratitude, abundance and generosity, you begin to harvest real sweetness in your life and let go of self-criticism. The more self-kindness I create, the less I desire sugary food.

Conversely, it is also essential to notice (but not fixate on) moments that grate. By allowing stronger emotions: anger, frustration or resentment to be acknowledged and released (your hypnosis recording helps so much with this because it restores feelings of calm, equanimity and forgiveness) you are actually reducing your desire for so called reward or comfort food. You are also protecting your heart, liver, gall bladder and kidneys….all organs that register the ill effects of negative thinking.

IMAGINE

Close your eyes for a moment and call to mind the most beautiful sunset imaginable. Perhaps you see golden clouds alight with the last rays of the day or maybe the sky is pink, lavender or aflame with orange. These colors remind you of your spirit and the majesty of life. The slights and frustrations of your day melt away in the presence of such beauty and you remember, instead, moments of sweetness, generosity and unexpected kindness. You feel blessed. You know that the enduring sweetness in life is an emotion and has nothing to do with food.

Affirmation:
"As I find new, healthier ways to nourish myself, I am grateful and content."

7. Enlighten Up!

Many of my wonderful students have told me that I should rename our class Enlighten Up because the process of creating a healthy relationship with food through hypnosis has opened their hearts and minds to a deeper spirituality. I believe that daily relaxation through hypnosis is similar to meditation and provides valuable spiritual nourishment. What we feed within grows. Hyp-

> Hypnosis feeds the spirit. Imagery is the language of the soul and hypnosis allows imagery to work in a powerful way to make change possible.

nosis feeds the spirit. Imagery is the language of the soul and hypnosis allows imagery to work in a powerful way to make change possible.

Billie joined *Lighten Up* class in the winter. At 5'5" her weight of 207 was an unhealthy burden. She was depressed and her physician had told her that she needed to lose weight. I knew right away that she had a problem with her thyroid and, indeed, this was confirmed and treated by an excellent CT endocrinologist.

Six months later, Billie now weighs 152 and is very close to her goal weight of 140. Billie is an "O" blood type and she readily adapted to the high protein, slow carbohydrate plan so ideal for "O"s. In addition to losing burdensome weight, Billy was delighted when her doctor was able to take her off of Zoloft and Wellbutrin for her depression had disappeared. Her digestion improved and she was also able to stop taking Zelnorm which was controlling symptoms of IBS. Billie loved self-hypnosis and learned how to put herself to sleep and to awaken at the designated time feeling refreshed. She no longer needed Ambien for insomnia and there were no more notes of tardiness or absenteeism at work. Her LDL cholesterol is now down by 30 points. She loves the energy and vitality she feels and is delighted by her new slender, youthful look.

Billie feels the greatest change has occurred in her spirit. She says "I was in a spiritual coma for over thirty years and now I am AWAKE !" Miraculously, when the body and spirit are BOTH nourished, feelings of balance, wellbeing and fulfillment triumph over frustration and despair. Billie has a new figure and a new lease on life. She is open to the spiritual vitality and goodness all around her. Her life is forever changed.

Alan, a successful engineer, discovered the importance of developing a kinder relationship with himself. Alan is a natural athlete who took high school football injuries in stride and maintained a healthy weight until his early thirties when a devastating car accident and subsequent spine injury grounded him and threatened his way of life. Alan is 6' 1" and his once lean, muscular body became burdened with excess weight during his long, slow recovery from back surgery. His surgeon told him that he would likely be confined to a wheelchair for the rest of his life. He gained nearly fifty pounds. Fortunately, with physical therapy and patience, Alan regained the use of his legs and he lost some of the weight. Up until the accident, Alan thought he was invincible. He continued to push himself very hard. Then, a few years later a severe knee injury led to more surgery and further weight gain. A healthy weight for Alan would be about 190.

When Alan joined my *Lighten Up* class he weighed 263. I remember his determination in that first class. He responded wonderfully to the *Lighten Up* plan and enjoyed eating for his "O" blood type which meant deleting wheat, dairy, peanuts and corn from his food choices and enjoying lean fish and meat, vegetables, fruit, walnuts and olive oil and Manna Bread (see resources). There were two aspects of hypnosis that truly helped him activate his will power: He discovered, while in hypnotic relaxation, that he truly DESERVED to take good care of himself and that he could let go of thinking that everybody and everything else had to come first. Secondly, he kept a photo of himself at his ideal, most fit ("ripped" in his words!) weight constantly in mind. His image of himself at his most healthy weight was the gateway to enduring will power.

Alan now weighs 215. His blood pressure and cholesterol levels are healthy and he will easily get to his goal weight of 190. He knows this healthy eating plan is not a diet but a way of life and he continues to listen to his Lighten Up recordings frequently. He knows that regular relaxation is not a luxury but a necessity.

IMAGINE

Recall a time when you felt love...unselfish, generous, unconditional love. Let this warm and radiant feeling expand in your awareness. Now see yourself as though YOU were your own dearest, most beloved friend and beam this radiance directly into your heart. Know that you truly deserve to be loved and to be well...now.

"As my body becomes more accustomed to regular exercise, I feel reserves of stored fat turning into lean muscle."

8.   The Skinny on Fat

I believe that our weight and cholesterol epidemic has more to do with excessive amounts of wheat and other refined carbohydrates (wheat is the biggest culprit) which tax the liver than with many fats. Folks in our *LU* classes who follow my caution against wheat flour products find they lose weight and that their cholesterol and triglyceride numbers improve significantly while waistlines diminish quickly. Moderate amounts of very lean meat and generous amounts of cold water fish provide excellent protein without elevating cholesterol.

> The body needs fat and some cholesterol but please know your fat

The body needs fat and some cholesterol but please know your fat: hydrogenated fat (solid like Crisco at room temperature) shows up in many foods you might consider to be wholesome such as commercial peanut butter. Nuts are very high in fat but contain only unsaturated fat, fiber, and protein which your body needs in appropriate amounts. A small amount (1/4 cup) of unsalted, unprocessed nuts is a good snack because you're having fat and fiber, both of which keep your blood sugar stable and satisfy your appetite. Nuts, olive oil, and flax oil actually help reduce the waistline as long as you don't overdo it. I keep walnuts and almonds in my desk because they help me stay slim and fit. I love them but I never eat more than a very small palm-full, and you shouldn't either.

Recent studies indicate that walnuts are prime, heart healthy fuel. The omega three fats in walnuts combined with fiber make them excellent food. Use caution with macadamia, pine, and cashew nuts for they have a very high fat to nutrition ratio.

Yes, olive oil is an excellent fat. You should buy extra virgin olive oil. But because it doesn't keep well (rancid oil is most unhealthy for your body) buy it in small amounts, use it up, and replenish it often. In addition to olive oil, you might also want to experiment with grape seed oil both in cooking and on salads. It is lighter than olive oil and full of powerful antioxidants.

Avocados are another source of beneficial, slimming fat and fiber. Here's a wonderful food that makes you glow, inside and out. Enjoy it sliced in salads or sandwiches or in your favorite guacamole dip. Because it combines fat and fiber, avocado is a wonderful food for satisfying your appetite and you'll love how its nutrients make your hair shine and your skin glow. It is truly a health and beauty food.

A fresh salad with healthy oil and lemon dressing is gorgeous and slimming. Add a few nuts for crunch or pumpkin seeds…no croutons please. The same salad with croutons and a creamy dressing is both fattening and toxic! It helps to really know what you are ingesting. Please say no thanks to creamy (ranch, blue cheese, Russian) dressings in favor of heart healthy olive oil based dressings. If you are eating in a restaurant, ask for your salad dressing on the side so that you are in charge of how much you eat. By the way, I love Paul Newman's balsamic dressing. He uses real olive oil, it is delicious, AND you'll be supporting his wonderful *Hole In The Wall Gang Foundation* which sponsors camping adventures for children with cancer

> Do you remember hearing someone say when you were a child that you should eat your fish because it is brain food. It's true! The brain absolutely must have these good omega 3 fats.

and other catastrophic illnesses. Riverlight Wellness Center supports this wonderful charity and its affiliate, *Angel Ride Foundation*, and I hope you will too.

A Miracle Fat

Fish Oil. Do you remember hearing someone say when you were a child that you should eat your fish because it is brain food. It's true! The brain absolutely must have these good omega 3 fatty acids. The health and waistline benefits of fresh, wild (therefore less toxic) cold water fish are also monumental. Fish, prepared in a simple and healthful way such as poached, broiled or baked, is a glorious protein source. If you are not a fish eater, it is important to take a very pure, pharmacy grade fish oil supplement regularly. Read supplement labels very carefully to be certain the oil has been filtered for toxins. You can purchase pharmacy grade fish oil quite easily now. Fish oil is a natural anti-depressant. It helps your immune system, your heart, and your joints and it makes your skin and hair glow. Try to get four to five servings of fresh, clean fish (avoid farm raised fish) into your weekly meals and enjoy the benefits of fish oil….a true youth elixir.

Another reason for eating fish liberally (no fried fish please) and taking supplements is that it is a natural anti-inflammatory food. The wonderful long chain fatty acids in omega 3 fish oil help reduce systemic inflammation in the body and may indeed hasten weight loss. I do wonder if small children who have been labeled inattentive in school wouldn't benefit from this marvelous oil in place of Ritalin for it truly helps quiet the mind and assist focus. Be a wise consumer and avoid all farm raised fish (salmon, cod, catfish are commonly farmed) as these fish have more toxins than wild fish and less nutrients because the feed they are given is inexpensive grain, loaded with food dyes and antibiotics. *A healthy tip,* canned sardines are an inexpensive and convenient supply of beneficial fish oil, protein, and calcium. They make a great snack or small meal. Canned wild Alaskan salmon is also a super food. Just add a little lemon, chopped celery and a teaspoon of mayonnaise and you've got a great tasting sandwich filling.

Flax is another valuable fat and fiber source. Ground flax (never cook it, for heat destroys its health benefits) is a precious anti-inflammatory food. Sprinkle two tablespoons on your morning cereal or add it to a smoothie. I put both flax and flax oil on my breakfast cereal with a little almond milk and blueberries....a great start to the day.

You'll find that when you eat foods that have both fat (the good kind) and fiber, you feel satisfied and you'll eat less. These beneficial fats: extra virgin olive oil, fish oil, nuts and nut oils, seeds (sunflower, pumpkin seeds), grape seed oil, and flax help your body metabolize stored belly fat. We truly need these nourishing fats to stay slim and disease free.

> Flax is another valuable fat and fiber source. Ground flax (never cook it, for heat destroys its health benefits) is a precious anti-inflammatory food.

Issues concerning food can be a metaphor for life issues. If you crave rich, fatty foods you may want to ask yourself if you tend to deny yourself life's richness and compensate by eating rich food instead. Can you call to mind five deliciously rich moments in your life that did not involve food? Hint: these might be moments of unexpected delight, tenderness, triumph, joy. If these rich moments are a scarcity in your life, perhaps it will help you to create some….that don't involve food. Just take time to appreciate a moment today when things were smooth, gentle or when a task was accomplished with ease. Remember what you focus on creates more of the same.

IMAGINE

In this moment, you can take a deep and generous breath and exhale all the irritations and discomforts you've been thinking about. You shift your awareness to all the moments when you felt at ease or when the Universe gave you a break. Your gratitude for those graceful moments of unexpected ease creates more and more moments of ease.

Affirmation:

"As I find new, healthier ways to nourish myself, I am grateful and content."

9. Got Milk?
You Might Need to Get Rid of It!!

If it comes from a cow, you might need to avoid it. The only way to find out if this is true for you is to eliminate all dairy from your meals for a week or two and notice if you feel better and any noticeable weight loss. If you have a tendency to get sinus infections or have allergies, you might benefit from a dairy cleanse. Worried about getting enough calcium? Enjoy

> Worried about getting enough calcium? Enjoy almonds, fresh spinach, sardines, broccoli, and take a calcium supplement. Your sinuses will love you for it!

almonds, fresh spinach, sardines, broccoli, and take a calcium supplement. Your sinuses will love you for it!

Another food on my hit list is American cheese. Wow, what an awful food and just think how many kids live on this. It is full of additives and food coloring, and it doesn't look or taste like real cheese. Putting cheese on meat is also a negative food choice if you are concerned about your weight and health. I know I'm bringing on the wrath of all the cheeseburger lovers out there. Sorry, please don't put cheese and meat together.

There are many excellent dairy substitutes on the market. You might like to try soy milk, cheese, and yogurt. Rice milk is good and I like almond milk. Goat and sheep milk, cheese, and yogurt tend to be easier to digest and cause less inflammation so you may want to try them.

Dr. Susan Lark (Women's Wellness Today Monthly Newsletter) contends that women over forty do not metabolize milk and other dairy products and I concur. So many diet plans revolve around large quantities of dairy (low fat milk, yogurt, cheese) but everyone is not alike and following mass dieting regimes backfires for many and leads to frustration. If you do eliminate dairy, you'll want to eat calcium rich foods and take a calcium supplement. Women absorb calcium best at night. Sardines, spinach and almonds are a few calcium rich foods.

If wheat and dairy are inflammatory foods for many of us, it isn't a surprise that our pizza-eating culture is heading toward its highest ever obesity rate. If you are like me, sensitive to wheat and dairy, a few slices of pizza will really have an uncomfortable impact on your body. Pizza in most cases is not a balanced meal for it contains too many carbs and calories, too much fat (not the good kind but saturated fat from the pepperoni and cheese), and not nearly enough vegetables and good quality protein. When trying to loose weight, please have a salad when your friends are eating pizza and if you're feeling deprived, ask for two meatballs but hold the cheese. Remember, there's no Morning After Pill for pizza … it is food but it isn't nourishment … it isn't FUEL.

IMAGINE

Close your eyes for a moment and imagine yourself feeling soothed and comforted. Expand these feelings of warmth and peace even more….float and drift in memories that calm you. When you are gentle with yourself, you won't feel the need for some of the creamy comfort foods that are unkind to your body. Mmmmmmmmmmmm.

"My body delights in the adventure of raw, wild, fiber filled food."

10.   Fabulous Fiber

Unfortunately, most of our food today is so over pro-cessed, our diets are woefully deficient in fiber. Fiber, especially when combined with a little beneficial fat (nuts, olive oil and seeds for example), really holds your appetite at bay. But beyond that, fiber is a natural anti-inflammatory food. Anyone with high cholesterol can usually improve quite rap-idly by adding more fiber to their diet. Flax and rice

> We need about 30 grams of fiber per day and most people don't get half that amount.

bran are two excellent sources of fiber. We need about 30 grams of fiber per day and most people don't get half that amount. Salads, raw fruit and vegetables, nuts and seeds and Manna bread (see resource list) are other high fiber foods. Most bran cereals also contain inflammatory amounts of wheat so I avoid those, but rice bran is won-derful. Reading food labels closely helps you see many so called fiber-rich breads and cereals just have added cellulose (a non dietary fiber…like eating tree bark but not as healthy as tree bark would be). Enjoy more and more foods with beneficial dietary fiber so your health will improve and your waistline will diminish. Fiber stimulates your metabolism and helps you maintain healthy blood sugar levels.

"More and more, as I notice all the sweetness around me, my appetite for sugary and fatty food lessens."

11.   Carbohydrates Decoded

There has certainly been a lot of misinformation about carbohydrates. Rest assured, the body needs carbs to function properly, but typical carb choices are making us fat: French fries, white rice, most bread, commercial pizza dough, and most brands of pasta. Choose carbs with a high fiber content and a low glycemic index—the rate at which the carb converts to sugar (which if unused is stored as body fat). For instance, the body perceives white rice/pasta/bread as equivalent to sugar. We've heard about low carb /high carb eating plans. The body benefits from SLOW CARBOHYDRATES, those that metabolize slowly: whole grains, legumes, vegetables, and fruit. Avoid all processed carbs: white sugar, pasta,

> Avoid all processed carbs: white sugar, pasta, ordinary wheat breads, desserts, and sweets. These stress the body and cause weight gain.

ordinary wheat breads, desserts, sweets, and mashed potatoes. These inflammatory foods stress the body and cause weight gain.

Positive Eating in Restaurants

Our love affair with potatoes has contributed to our tight waistbands. Nearly every restaurant mounds mashed potatoes (loaded with butter, cream…ouch!) or French fries on your plate along with the main course. Well sure, potatoes are far less expensive and easier to prepare and reheat (they have a longer shelf life) than fresh vegetables. This trend is killing us…add a cocktail or two, a basketful of white bread with butter and a rich dessert and we have a health disaster in the making. Your bathroom scale will register this assault. A recent Harvard study indicated that people who eat large quantities of potatoes, especially mashed and fried, are more likely to develop Type II Diabetes symptoms. Cut back on white potatoes and enjoy sweet potatoes, squash and full fiber whole grains.

As an empowered, knowledgeable diner, you must ask for the food you need and ask your waiter to help you adapt the menu offerings to benefit and nourish you. When I go out for a meal, I order fish or lean meat (no sauces, breading or heaven forbid, deep fat frying), no potatoes (the exception being sweet potatoes and they don't need any butter) and extra vegetables, preferably steamed. If it is a special occasion, I might have one glass of good red wine with my meal. Tell your waiter to take the bread away. This is YOUR meal and YOU are paying for it so please give yourself permission to make the requests that benefit you.

High value carbohydrates include: fresh fruit, fresh vegetables, baked sweet potatoes, whole grain brown rice, legumes (chick peas, black beans, adzuki beans, black eyed peas) to name a few. Enjoy fruit whole, the skin has valuable fiber and vitamins. Commercial fruit juice is not a beneficial food. By the time it gets to you it has lost much of its nutrient benefit and it is intensely sugary with a high carbohydrate value...

> High value carbohydrates include: fresh fruit, fresh vegetables, baked sweet potatoes, whole grain brown rice, legumes (chick peas, black beans, adzuki beans, black eyed peas) to name a few.

have the whole fruit just as nature intended. So, if you begin your day with a large glass of commercial orange juice, you are drinking a sugary, low value carbohydrate which raises your blood sugar and primes your appetite for more sugar. Have a whole orange or grapefruit instead. If you have a juicer at home, you are getting a very high quality juice but without the fruit's precious fiber which helps you metabolize carbs!

Fresh vegetable juices are wonderful supplements to your meal plan. A glass of freshly prepared green juice is a great in between meal snack—celery, spinach...with a bit of apple is very refreshing and brimming with nutrients. Or try a glass of freshly prepared green juice at the start of your meal…it will take the edge off your appetite and you'll be satisfied eating less. If you don't have a juicer, there are a wide variety of green juice products which are very low in calories and carbs and very high in nutritive value: Perfect Food, Barleens, Sun Chlorella, to name a few. Please add a green juice food to your daily diet. Your skin, hair, eyes, mood and waistline will love you for it and so will your blood pressure! And by the way, V-8 juice doesn't count…it is too processed and too high in sodium to be a beneficial food for you, wonderful you! Green vegetables help us metabolize saturated and trans fats. As you get more greens into your diet, your weight will naturally decrease.

Our excessive appetite for bread, pasta, and noodles is exacerbating our national obesity trend. If you've traveled in Italy, you've discovered that pasta is only a small part of the meal which includes vegetables, olive oil, and fish or meat. Here we make pasta the main course; we pile our plate sky high with this over-used carb and then douse

> Our excessive appetite for bread, pasta, and noodles is exacerbating our national obesity trend.

it with meat sauce, cheese or both…spaghetti night!! This kind of meal is an assault on your body, for it simply can't metabolize this many carbs combined with colossal amounts of fat. Add several servings of white bread and butter, extra cheese and you've put yourself in the danger zone.

I love pasta but I no longer eat wheat based pasta. If we're having pasta, I prepare rice pasta and serve it sparingly with a homemade red sauce (lots of chopped vegetables so it is nothing like the sauce that comes in a jar) or pesto or garlic and olive oil...and here's the important part...the portion is small...not a mound but about a cup of pasta with a cup of sauce. The rest of the meal consists of a lush green salad dressed with olive oil and garlic bread made with olive oil, garlic, herbs on Manna bread and a glass of red wine. Dessert might be fresh berries and a small wheat free oatmeal cookie (see Resources for recipe).

Since you can't usually get rice based pasta in restaurants, I suggest you avoid pasta in favor of lean meat or fish but if you must, ask for a half portion and don't bury it in cheese, say no thank you to the bread and enjoy a large salad with olive oil based dressing...no cream (ranch) or cheese (Roquefort) based dressings for your glorious body! Remember, when you go for the good fats, it helps you get rid of your spare tire. If you are a vegetarian, choose pasta with lots of vegetables and sautéed tofu. Do try to eat pastas made from quinoa or rice as these are less inflammatory than wheat based pastas and they taste delicious. As you know, beans and rice make a complete protein so choose healthy combinations and be cautious with cheese toppings and sauces for they can be loaded with fat and calories. A pasta topping of fresh vegetables sautéed in garlic and extra virgin olive oil makes a great meal…add a little sautéed tofu for some vegetable protein.

A word about rice…a cup of white rice is equivalent to a cup of white sugar as far as your body knows. Most Chinese food is served with white rice (and Indian food), but you might as well ask for a serving of sugar with your lamb curry or your egg foo yong. White rice is a better bet than pasta if you are sensitive to wheat (and most of us are) but it needs to be served with lots of fibrous vegetables and good fat in order for your body to metabolize it without a huge rise in blood sugar. Avoid it if you can and if not, small amounts, please.

Good quality, whole grain brown rice is a terrific food. A low glycemic index carb, it satisfies your appetite. A cup of cooked rice is a reasonable portion. Add it to soups or stews and enjoy it often. It keeps well so you can make a batch for the week, reheating it or serving it with stir fry or whatever the menu calls for.

Quinoa is a miracle grain which you cook just like rice. It boasts fiber, protein, amino acids and omega 3 fats. Try adding it to soups or serving it in place of rice. In addition to the grain, you can purchase quinoa flour and flakes. Use these in place of wheat flour in your baking for a delicious and more nutritious end result.

Affirmation:
"Breakfast is a daily celebration: I begin my day with a nutrient rich meal which sustains me."

12. Meals In Detail

Now that you've gotten this far, I'd like to review some points and expand a bit on meal planning for the entire day. Let me emphasize again, breakfast is your most important meal of the day.....NEVER, NEVER, NEVER, skip breakfast if you are trying to lose weight. Until you've hydrated well (remember, 16 oz. of water when you wake up) and eaten a meal consisting of protein, good fat, and beneficial carbohydrates, your metabolic switch is off.

Let's talk about breakfast cereals. Simply put, if it comes in a box, it is most likely too processed to be of value to you. Most commercial breakfast cereals are loaded with sugar, wheat, and a whole host of other additives. They are high in carbohydrates and low on nutrients. And granola can be worse for it is often loaded with sugar. Cereals that really nourish you are: oats (preferably the whole oat groat...just as nature intended), rye, quinoa, and kamut. These whole grains can be cooked ahead of time...you prepare them like rice, and you can make a week's worth and refrigerate.

Add ground flax and a bit of flax oil to cooked cereal (don't cook flax products for this destroys their beneficial omega oils) and top with skim milk, soy, rice, or almond milk. Add a small handful of nuts and fresh fruit (1/2 banana or some fresh berries) and you have a satisfying, fiber-filled breakfast. Remember, when you add fat and fiber to a meal or snack, your appetite will be satisfied for a longer time.

Eggs make a great breakfast if they are properly prepared. Eggs have gotten a bad rap because they do contain cholesterol. In moderation, they are a perfect food as long as you don't overcook the yolk. Scrambled eggs, omelets, and hardboiled eggs have an imbalance of cholesterol because the yolk's precious lecithin (a natural emulsifier) is destroyed when the yolk is cooked. But a soft boiled, poached, or over-easy (easy on the fat in the pan...spray on olive oil is best) egg is a good protein source for you because it won't elevate your cholesterol unless you eat wheat based bread or bacon with it. En-

Adding a cup or two of green tea to your breakfast is a great way of boosting your metabolism. Green tea is full of antioxidants but, more importantly for slenderizing, it has thermogenic qualities which help your metabolism function at a higher rate.

joy organic eggs. I buy the smallest size eggs I can get, avoiding extra large eggs for those come from older chickens. You can buy free-range eggs in most grocery stores and these really are best.

Adding a cup or two of green tea to your breakfast is a great way of boosting your metabolism. Green tea is full of antioxidants but, more importantly for slenderizing, it has thermogenic qualities which help your metabolism function at a higher rate. Authentic green tea leaves look green after brewing. If the leaves seem dark and brownish, change your brand until you see green tea leaves and then you'll know you have the real thing. Steep briefly or it can become quite bitter. If you need sweetening, sprinkle a little stevia into your tea. Stevia is a plant that is sweeter than sugar yet safe for diabetics. It tends to decrease your sugar cravings. Please make green tea a part of your wellbeing plan.

Take green tea to work with you and enjoy it instead of coffee. While coffee is stimulating, green tea contains the amino acid L-theanine which is very calming to the mind.

Affirmation:
"I plan ahead so I always have just the right food. I deserve only the best."

13. Food for the Workday

Office Celebrations

Many people start their day with a positive attitude about food but then all their good intentions fall apart on the job for the workplace is full of saboteurs! Every coffee cake, birthday cake, leftover pie, candy, and cookie (and don't even get me started on danish and doughnuts) is a potential trap. I'm amazed by how many CEOs there are who come to me for

> Make sure you have a good plan for lunch so you don't get caught in the pizza/burger/taco takeout nightmare.

weight loss assistance and tell me they feel tyrannized by all the food people bring to the office. The great thing about being in charge is that you can easily put a stop to this. Organize a fruit basket instead. Encourage staff to celebrate either with healthy food and snacks or without them. Bring your own fruit/nuts/healthy snack to work so you can join in on the celebration but not the tyranny. You're wonderful and you deserve to take a break, but you don't deserve coffee cake....you're much too precious for that.

Lunch

Make sure you have a good plan for lunch so you don't get caught in the pizza/burger/taco takeout nightmare. Perhaps there's a place nearby where you can get soup and salads that are freshly made and full of lovely vegetables and lean protein. A green salad with a bit of protein is great, but insist on olive oil based dressing and put your own on...just a drizzle will do. Say "no thank you" to croutons...instead add nuts, pumpkin seeds, and lots of celery for crunch and fiber.

If the take-out options near your workplace don't meet your needs, then take the extra time to prepare lunch for yourself to take to work with you. You're worth it!!

Snacks

You may want to take a healthy afternoon snack to work too so you get through the afternoon without running out of steam. An apple, some nuts perhaps or a rice cracker with nut butter are all easy to manage. This is a really good time to have a green drink; it will perk you up in a healthy way (unlike coffee or caffeinated sodas) and get another nutrient rich vegetable serving into your system. The important thing is to manage your hunger—avoid becoming ravenous and therefore out of control. If you are someone who eats thoughtfully and sparingly all day but spins out of control in the late afternoon or evening, circumvent this tendency by having a vegetable drink or snack in the late afternoon. And don't forget water.....lots and lots of water.

"Each day, I move my body more and more, and I find that being active creates energy reserves I can feel."

14. Metabolism

For most people, the food eaten after 5:00 PM (and beverage consumed) is either a weight loss benefit or culprit. As we get older, our metabolism slows down and when we don't make adjustments, weight will pile on. I have a friend who is now in her 70s and she continues to lament that when she was younger she could eat bread, pasta, fried food, and desserts and never gain an ounce. She was considered a skinny kid, a very thin adult, and now is an overweight senior. Her metabolism has slowed down but she hasn't adjusted her consumption. Sugary, caloric cocktails, large dinners, and desserts have caused her to gain weight. Sore joints make her reluctant to exercise. Sound familiar?

I confess that I've gone through a number of metabolic shifts in my life. The one I remember most vividly occurred around the time of my 30th birthday. Up until that time, my weight had never been a concern except in the months following two pregnancies when I managed to look pregnant AFTER delivering because of weight gain.

Anyway, in those days my favorite meal was steamed Maine clams, lobster (yes, butter!), French fries (they say confession is good for the soul!!), and pecan pie with whipped cream. We lived on an island in Maine and a big night out with two little ones in tow consisted of a boat trip across the bay to a favorite lobster restaurant. The summer of my 30th year brought forth the rude awakening that I couldn't zip up my jeans and keep eating this way. I learned to delete the butter and French fries; I added a green salad with a vinaigrette dressing, allowed myself three bites of pie, and managed to get back into my jeans. As my metabolism changed, I adjusted my eating and exercise habits accordingly.

The point of this story is that we have to recognize our own metabolic shifts and adjust. I believe that naturally thin people do this automatically. Instead of buying a larger size wardrobe when they gain a few pounds, they take the weight off instead and manage to keep a healthy weight balance. Please don't be like my friend …clinging to the memory of a skinny childhood while her senior body sends signals that it is time to recognize where her metabolism is now and to cut back on all the desserts.

How to Push Your Metabolic Set Point Up a Few Notches So You Can Easily Lose Weight

I believe that we can enhance and support metabolism to get its optimal benefit and sustain healthy weight BUT…this takes consistent effort.

Start your day with 16 oz of *water* and keep hydrating all day (except during meals).

Avoid all sugar substitutes (except for stevia which seems to quiet sugar cravings).

Eat breakfast…this first meal of the day engages your metabolism. Breakfast eaters are less likely to be over eaters.

Don't skip meals and avoid becoming ravenously hungry…have a green drink!

For every decade you've lived, your body needs ten minutes a day of aerobic exercise (running, brisk walking, biking)…

Exercise!! For every decade you've lived, your body needs ten minutes a day of exercise (running, brisk walking, biking) so if you are 40, you need to exercise for a minimum of 40 minutes per day…every day because your body doesn't know the difference between Tuesday and Saturday. So get moving. If you haven't been exercising, start slowly, but make this 10 minute per decade equation your goal and work up to it slowly but with commitment! In addition to your 10 minutes per decade (if you're 49, round upward to

50 minutes per day), you will need to do some weight bearing exercise three days per week. As you convert fat to lean muscle, your metabolism will shift and you will be able to restore your calorie burning capability.

Did you know that every time you lose muscle (most dieting causes this...especially yo-yo dieting) you decrease your calorie burning capability? This is one of the ways that dieting makes us fat. Every ounce of muscle lost during each weight loss episode in your life is stored in your metabolic memory bank and it shrinks your body's capacity to utilize subsequent calories. In other words, your sluggish metabolism may be paying now for past dieting consequences. The only way to reverse this is with an active muscle building program. This is why exercise is so crucial.

Get at least 7 hours of sleep. Your body replenishes and renews itself during restful sleep but it also does its hardest metabolic work while you are sleeping. Slender bodies are well rested bodies.

Fast...don't eat after supper until breakfast. Ideally 11 hours without food will elapse from your last meal in the evening until breakfast the next morning. Your metabolism needs this "down time" to do its work.

Breathe deeply often! You can't imagine how this activates your metabolism. Four slow deep breaths which really focus on the exhale can reignite your metabolism, not to mention lower your blood pressure and your cortisol stress hormone levels. Do this often throughout the day...at your desk, while sitting in traffic or waiting in line at the store.

> Four slow deep breaths which really focus on the exhale can reignite your metabolism, not to mention lower your blood pressure and your cortisol stress hormone levels. Do this often throughout the day.

Drink green tea. There's plenty of evidence that green tea, which is loaded with antioxidants, has a thermogenic effect. In other words it heats up your metabolism. If you want to lose weight, switch from coffee to green tea. Your blood pressure and your waistline will thank you.

Take breaks and exercise a little bit...a five minute brisk walk (easy to accomplish if you park your car a short walk from your destination), or if there are stairs in your building, go up and down them a few times, often. When I lived in London my flat was on the fourth floor and although we had a lift (elevator), I always took the stairs. So three or four times a day I got this little extra boost to my metabolism. When I would return to Connecticut and step on the scale, my weight was always a few pounds lighter. See if you can find new opportunities to add little bursts of effort to your day and watch your weight drop.

A great time to get a little extra motion into your life is while watching TV. My *Lighten Up* students get a laugh out of watching me demonstrate the following but it will change your life and your weight. If you are a TV fan, *plan to exercise during those annoying TV ads.* Have 1 or 2 lb hand weights nearby and during the dreaded ad, stand and then sit down while lifting the weights at a 90 degree angle (modified squats) as you stand and sit. If there are 2-minute commercials every 15 minutes, you might add as much as 8–10 minutes of weight bearing exercise while watching an hour of TV. If you don't have weights (but you will want to get some) use two cans of soup! And keep sipping from that water bottle.

Affirmation:

"It is fun and exciting to exercise regularly, and I enjoy getting stronger."

15. Get Moving, Get Gorgeous

There are certain habits that naturally thin people practice that you can incorporate into your life. One thing is just to move more. Just simply move your arms and legs more, and more often. Set small tasks or goals for yourself that involve movement and then reward yourself (but not with food) for accomplishing them. Your conscious awareness of how much sitting you do and how much motion you choose is crucial to your success. Avoid all shortcuts that

As you gradually convert stored fat to lean muscle, you not only look, feel, and function better, you actually increase your body's capability to utilize the calories you eat more efficiently.

reduce the time you spend moving…stairs are great, walking is good, carrying things works your arms and shoulders. You might write out a list of regular chores and tasks and see if there is a way you can get more motion into their completion. Think of this as a way you choose to be GENEROUS with yourself.

Exercise has so many benefits, not the least of which is the way it reduces soreness, aches and pains, because when you exercise you help release lactic acid from your muscles (toxic when it doesn't get released). Your body also releases delightful endorphins during and after exercise which create feelings of wellbeing and reduction of discomfort. So when you feel achy and stiff, exercise IS the best medicine.

As you gradually convert stored fat to lean muscle, you not only look, feel, and function better, you actually increase your body's capability to utilize the calories you eat more efficiently. Some people enjoy wearing a pedometer just to see how many real steps they take each day. I had one weight loss client who insisted she "ran her feet off" every day and didn't need to exercise. At my request, she wore a pedometer (you can buy them for as little as $1.00) and discovered that she was only taking 900 steps per day. She gradually worked up to 10,000 steps (five miles) and is now a vision of health and vitality.

Start your walking plan gradually and ALWAYS check with your doctor first before you begin an exercise program. If you've been sedentary, try for 2,000 steps per day and increase each week by increments of 500 steps. As you walk, deliberately accelerate the pace for a minute or two and then decrease, accelerate again for 3 minutes and then slow down…this form of pulse exercise helps activate your metabolism and it is a great way to get a walking program working for your wonderful friend, your body!

Beware of any weight loss program that doesn't emphasize exercise because it is doomed to fail. Just know as you listen to your hypnosis recording, your resistance to exercising regularly and joyfully will melt away. Remember, hypnosis helps you change your mind about long-held beliefs and break through barriers of resistance. Your subconscious mind remembers all the times you felt relaxed, free and comfortable in your body. It remembers how much you enjoyed playing (exercising) when you were young. Let

> What is the best form of exercise? Whatever form that you can enjoy and commit to.

hypnosis assist you in recalling such memories. They can be the basis of your commitment to exercise often and well as you consistently release sedentary patterns…and watch a slender you emerge.

What is the best form of exercise? Whatever form that you can enjoy and commit to. Many exercise attempts fail because, without commitment, our desires just become wishful thinking. If you hate going to the gym, you are unlikely to be successful exercising that way. Dancing is a wonderful way to share exercise time with a friend or partner. Walking is always a good choice, especially if you are just beginning your exercise program. If you are sociable, you might enjoy taking a fitness, yoga, or Pilates class, and spinning is one workout that really revs your metabolism and burns fat. If exercise is also a form of recreation that is enjoyable (like tennis, golf, skiing, or neighborhood basketball) you will be more likely to stick to it.

Exercise is also fuel…it fuels your energy bank. Just take a walk the next time you feel tired at the end of the day and notice that you feel better and more alert. Get the energy you need through regular exercise. When you combine that with moderate, nourishing meals, healthy sleep, and the rest and rejuvenation you get from your hypnosis recording, you'll start to feel like a new person. Exercise raises beta-endorphins which create delightful sensations of relaxation, calm and ease.

Personal Power and Weight

Unexpended energy or inertia often leads to weight gain. You may have noticed that the most dynamic people in your sphere consider regular exercise an important part of life. Each of us has a personal power point. This is a place just beyond what we consider comfortable exertion. If you've ever worked with a personal trainer you know that he or she endeavors to inspire you to find this point. It is NOT about injuring yourself or over-riding your body's wisdom. It may be a place where you can excel. It is a breath beyond what you think you can do (walk for another fifteen minutes) and what you CAN do.

Very dynamic people need to fully inhabit their "power point place" to be completely healthy. Exercise is one of the ways this happens. Think, for a moment, of a celebrated athlete and how charismatic (Tiger Woods, the Williams sisters, Lance Armstrong) they are. This charisma comes from more than mere personality. When we exercise into and beyond resistance, we build personal power. This is a kind of inner radiance and confidence that shines brightly in the world like the Olympic flame.

A great example of this principal in action is Oprah. We know that she was challenged by her weight for years and through many, many weight loss cycles. Her diet history is well documented. We loved her regardless of her weight. She is now healed for she is truly living her power and radiance. Oprah affirms and claims her absolute right to this by lifting weights and challenging her body to be as powerful and strong as her spirit and persona is. A little gentle yoga (lovely and healthful as it is) would not fully express the energetic being of Oprah. Her central theme is strength and radiance and her primary exercise expresses this. Through living her power fully, Oprah has finally attained and maintained a healthy weight. She is living her body's truth by loving and practicing the discipline and challenge of strength training.

Are you a dancer or a marathoner at heart? What aspect of your own personal power have you denied? What is YOUR inner truth about what your body wishes to express? When you discover the full dimension of your inner power, you'll find it easier to achieve and maintain a healthy weight. Often this aspect is the very part of ourselves that we've been most afraid of but once it is discovered and freely brought forth, joy prevails. Do you think Oprah likes this newly developed strength? Of course she does!

Power is very, very personal. It may be action or stillness. It may be the ability to use your voice and sing your deepest song. You may write, marathon, advocate, lead or create something wild and raw. Find your radiance, welcome it and live it fully. You won't regret it. To do this, perhaps you'll need to release old thought forms. A parent or sibling may have scolded you into silence or demanded you sit still (don't draw attention to yourself) and food may have been part of this disempowering process. Still, you can decide to live your power now. The world needs you to live out loud and at full radiance.

Say yes!

IMAGINE

You are a radiant beam of light. What color are you?
How much light do you generate and hold within? If
you were a generator, how would your vast reserves of
energy be deployed to make your life better and better?
How much more active would you like to be? Picture
yourself joyfully, wildly active and loving it. Celebrate
all that is within you and let it shine forth.

Affirmation:
"I know when I relax and take a few deep breaths, my metabolism improves and my mood lightens."

16. Mood and Weight

One of the ways we are overmedicated in this country is the prolific use of anti–depressants. I believe that they may be directly related to weight gain. Please don't stop taking your medication! However, if you are heavier than you or your doctor would like you to be and you are taking antidepressants, please read my friend Gracelyn Guyol's wonderful book: *Healing Depression and Bipolar Disorder Without Drugs.* Most mood disorders are a form of malnutrition. When your brain gets the fuel it needs, it functions well. When it doesn't, it registers its starvation by making you feel depressed, moody and unfocused.

> When your brain gets the fuel it needs, it functions well. When it doesn't, it registers its starvation by making you feel depressed, moody and unfocused.

One top form of brain fuel is Omega 3 Fish Oil. Most people don't take enough of it to get the greatest benefit from it. Most adults benefit from 4 grams daily. For someone who has lots of inflammation or who is suffering from depression, it might be of benefit to take up to 6 grams of fish oil per day until the mood lightens. This miracle food helps you stay focused and calm and creates feelings of balance and wellbeing. Omega 3 long-chain fatty acids used to be much more prevalent in our diets when agriculture used fish emulsion as fertilizer. Now so many of our fertilizers are simply chemicals which produce less nutritious food. If you don't eat fish regularly, you'll want to add pure, filtered, fish oil to your daily fuel. Note: If you take other blood thinners—prescription anticoagulants, garlic, ginko, or aspirin—be sure to speak with your doctor before adding Omega 3 oils to your diet.

When you visit my web site (www.riverlightcenter. com) to download your free hypnosis recording, you'll have a chance to learn about Brain State Technology TM, an innovative brain balancing system that helps alleviate depression, anxiety and cravings of all sorts. There may be a qualified BST TM trainer near you who will help you achieve optimal brain balance and harmony in a pleasant and non-invasive way.

Affirmation:

"I bless the children in my life with the joys of fresh, life-giving food and the pleasure of regular, playful exercise.""

17. Lighten Up Our Kids!

Sadly, the most overfed, undernourished and overmedicated in our population are our children. Childhood obesity rates are soaring. Children with allergies and poor immune systems fail to thrive in school and many suffer the terrible stigma of being overweight.

Many children subsist on processed, poor quality food. It is difficult to find a school lunch menu that features adequate amounts of protein (essential for healthy brain function), healthy fat, slow carbohydrates, vitamins and minerals. Compound this with the fact that many children do not get enough daily fresh fruit

Did you ever invite a child to bend down and pluck a juicy, sweet strawberry?

and vegetables and it is no wonder that so many of our precious youngsters are faltering.

I salute Michelle Obama's initiatives aimed at ending childhood obesity and I laud her example of creating a

White House garden. I am hopeful that her efforts will have a long term impact on family health awareness. Perhaps you'll plant a simple garden in your back yard, in containers on your deck or patio or at your windowsill. Many towns have community garden plots and urban gardeners create ingenious roof-top vegetable gardens.

Have you ever taken a child into a vegetable garden and invited her to pick a ripe, fat peapod and gobble up its sweet contents? Did you ever invite a child to bend down and pluck a juicy, sweet strawberry? My two year old granddaughter ate raw asparagus and peas in her ninety year old great-grandfather's garden last summer. The look of delight on her face (and her discovery that her favorite foods actually have an origin other than the grocery store or the freezer) made this simple summer pleasure a precious memory. Her favorite food is fresh, sweet corn and when we go to the farm to get our corn, she hugs the corn stalks in gratitude. Children have a natural affinity for gardens and they'll usually eat raw vegetables right from the garden....they can't resist.

Even if you don't have a garden, you can guide the children in your life away from low-value foods. Healthy eating starts at the beginning of life. Mother's milk is perfect food for the first six months of life. It is full of nourishment and immunity (colostrum in mother's milk protects newborns) boosters. Both mother and baby benefit from the loving, trust building connection breastfeeding affords.

I am very concerned about the quality of store bought milk and its effect on the health of our children. Believe me, what's found in containers on your grocery shelf bears very little resemblance to its original form. Please buy organic milk if you can and do know that after the age of one or so, large amounts of dairy are problematic for healthy children. First, children fill up on milk and are less likely to eat a more balanced meal. Second, the cows milk that most children consume is a very poor rendition of its original self due to over processing and additives. Children are fed way too many processed cheese products as well (American Cheese is a toxic, processed substance and should not be considered viable food). Children who have chronic colds and respiratory infections usually benefit from a reduction or elimination of dairy foods. Check with your pediatrician if this is a concern.

Some prepared baby food is certainly better than the nasty tasting, over-salted jarred variety available when my children were babies. I made all my own baby food (often from our garden) by using a baby food grinder and adapting our meals to feed everyone. Roast chicken, beef stew with fresh vegetables, brown rice, fresh raw apples, pears and peaches (organic please, too many pesticides in the non-organic variety) were all easily ground up and served to baby. A baked, mashed sweet potato is wonderful baby food as is mashed banana and avocado. Quinoa flakes make a delightful first cereal.

Just as wheat is an inflammatory food for adults, it is also inflamatory for children. Avoiding wheat based cereals is certainly a good idea. Children need a great breakfast: quinoa, oat or rice cereal, a soft-boiled egg, toast with pure nut butter and fresh fruit all help a young body and mind to thrive and do well in school. Please don't give sugary processed cereals to children no matter how much they beg for them!

My granddaughter absolutely loves avocado and we find it easy to slice a ripe one in half and feed her right from the "avocado boat" as she calls it. Or perhaps your youngster might like freshly made guacamole with baked (not fried) whole grain chips. Steamed green beans or broccoli florets (please buy organic when you can, green beans are on the top of the excessive use of pesticide lists) appeal to children who like finger foods.

You can buy frozen sweet potato french fries and they are a wonderful alternative to the unhealthy white potato version. Or you can make your own health "fries" by slicing a washed, unpeeled sweet potato and baking it in a well oiled (olive oil, please) pan until crisp. Hand a child a steamed ear of summer sweet corn (no need for butter) and watch it disappear.

We make quinoa cakes for snacks and meals. Add two beaten eggs to one cup of cooked grain that you have cooled. You can include chopped parsley, cilantro, onion or garlic and then sauté the mixture (about two tablespoons per cake) in olive oil. The cooked cakes freeze well and are easily reheated. These crunchy and flavorful cakes are packed with nutrition ideal for children: protein, fiber, amino acids, and brain healthy fatty acids. Grownups love them, too!

See how you can adapt foods from the Miracle Food list in the next chapter to appeal to the children in your life. Introduce raw foods to young children: blueberries, raw peas and beans, apples, and sprouts are all appealing to many children.

Just as exercise is crucial in attaining a healthy weight for adults, children also need to get plenty of exercise and fresh air. Too many of our children sit in school all day (many schools have cut back on gym classes and outdoor activity) and then go home and sit in front of a television set or computer. It is no wonder that many children experience disturbed sleep and difficulty concentrating in school. Parents and adult family members must set a better example. If your children see you collapse on the couch after work, they will grow up to do the same thing. Let's get our kids moving, playing and enjoying garden fresh foods.

One last thing: habits that begin in early childhood often persist with negative results into adulthood. In my hypnosis practice, I work with many who have food addictions that stem from early childhood. Often fussy children are placated with sugary foods and fattening substitutes for real human comfort. Kids who get a cookie or candy to distract from the pain of a skinned knee or an upset often grow up to use food as distraction from emotional or physical pain. Please hug, hold, soothe and comfort your distressed children but don't give them sweets for comfort.

Affirmation:
"I enjoy trying new foods and experiencing new textures, flavors, colors."

18. Miracle Foods

Miracle Foods that help us get well and stay well:
Fish Oil (use with a doctor's supervision if taking blood thinning medicines)

Flax oil and ground flax seed (never expose to heat, cooking and baking destroys vital nutrients)

Blueberries

Celery (very purifying and a natural diuretic)

Asparagus: (kidney cleanse, diuretic)

Dark chocolate (a tiny portion of 70% or more cocoa)

Red wine (in moderation)

Almonds (full of zinc, calcium and a natural blood thinner)

Sweet potatoes: (full of fiber and vitamin A)

Artichokes (full of fiber and alkalizing)

Cruciferous vegetables: broccoli, brussels sprouts, cauliflower

Avocado: (beneficial fats, wonderful for glowing skin)

Kelp: a thyroid-nourishing sea weed

Parsley: (a cleansing, cooling, green food)

Wild salmon: (full of omega 3 fish oil)

Sardines: (full of calcium and omega 3s)

Walnuts: (fiber and omega 3 oil)

Dark grapes: (antioxidants and potassium)

Collards and kale: (highest nutrient content of all green leafy veggies)

Quinoa grain and flour (protein, omega 3 fats, fiber, amino acids)

Salba grain (amino acids, protein, fiber, beneficial fats)

Açai juice (antioxidants, omega fats)

Enjoy the adventure of adding new foods to your meals!

Affirmation:
"When I take a moment to focus my mind on success, the results are powerful."

19. Step by Step Self-Hypnosis

Change your mind now about food and exercise
In less time than it takes you to wash your hands, you can easily program yourself to eat less, to make positive food choices and to exercise more—three habits combined that will help you achieve and maintain a healthy weight.

In addition to listening to your *Lighten Up! Win At Losing* recording each day (remember it lowers your cortisol, thus helping you lose belly fat) you'll want to practice self-hypnosis which will super charge your will power reserves

> In less time than it takes you to wash your hands, you can easily program yourself to eat less, to make positive food choices and to exercise more

and place the POWER of your sub-conscious mind in your hands.

Self-Hypnosis Step by Step

Begin by sitting comfortably in a chair with spine straight and feet on the floor.

1. Take a few deep breaths and focus on your exhale.

2. Keeping your chin at a 90 degree angle (not up or down…just natural), raise your eyes toward the ceiling and then close your eyelids…breathe…and repeat this 5 times.

3. Now, with your eyes open, bring your dominant hand up toward your face just in front of your eyes. Focus your eyes on the tips of your index finger and thumb which are about 2 inches apart.

4. Still focusing on your finger tips, count silently downwards from 5 to 1 and when you get to one, the pointer and thumb touch. Close your eyes and rub your finger tips together (you are creating an anchoring signal in your body).

5. Now let your arm drift slow-motion style down toward your body…it should feel very slow, very relaxing and good.

6. Silently state your self-hypnosis statement over and over five times and see yourself enacting these desired behaviors and results.

7. Count up from 1 to 5, and on 5, once more rub thumb and pointer finger tips together and let your eyes open. You have successfully programmed your healthy food and exercise choices.

Affirmation:
"I eat less, exercise more, and enjoy healthy changes in my body and my life."

20. Affirmations for Healthy, Lasting Weight Loss

- I eat less, exercise more and enjoy healthy changes in my body and my life.

- I choose high value foods, eat less and feel satisfied and nourished.

- More and more, as I notice all the sweetness around me, my appetite for sugary and fatty food lessens.

- I take time each day to picture myself at a healthy weight; feeling and looking wonderful and this picture of me guides my actions and choices.

- It is fun and exciting to exercise regularly and I enjoy getting stronger.

- Each day, I move my body more and more and I find that being active creates energy reserves I can feel.

- As my body becomes more accustomed to regular exercise, I feel reserves of stored fat turning into lean muscle.

- I know that when I relax and take a few deep breaths, my metabolism improves and my mood lightens.

- I am doing well and I enjoy turning old cravings into healthy actions.

- I listen closely and deeply to the messages and needs of my body and nourish it thoughtfully.

- More and more I enjoy fresh, wholesome, colorful, energy giving food.

- As I find new, healthier ways to nourish myself, I am grateful and content.

- My body delights in the adventure of raw, wild, fiber filled food.

- Breakfast is a daily celebration: I begin my day with a nutrient rich meal which sustains me.

- I plan ahead so I always have just the right food. I deserve only the best.

- I enjoy trying new foods and experiencing new textures, flavors, colors.

- When I take a moment to focus my mind on success, the results are powerful.

Choose one affirmation that feels right to you and make it your mantra.

21. Resources

Dr. Peter D'Adamo, *4Your Blood Type* books and Blood typing kit: www.4yourbloodtype.com

Dr. Theodore Baroody, *Alkalize or Die,* a compelling book on the value of alkaline balance for healthy weight

Shopping notes: Manna bread products (in the frozen food section of most grocery stores). Manna bread is made from all sprouted grains and is less inflammatory than standard wheat-based bread products.

Mary's Gone Crackers: a crisp, delicious non-wheat cracker

Food For Life: Almond Rice Bread (gluten free)

I have not included many recipes in this book because I want you to move away from the idea of recipes since most have unhealthy consequences. However, I'm including two recipes here to help you get started. If you focus on meals that consist of a small amount of lean protein and generous portions of freshly picked vegetables and fruits and thoughtfully selected grains, you will thrive.

Walnut Butter: An excellent way to add brain-healthy fat and fiber to your diet:
1 ½ cup walnut pieces
¼ cup of fresh walnut oil (or flax oil)
¼ cup ground flax or ground salba
A pinch of sea salt

Chop nuts in food processor until fine, add salt, ground flax (or salba), drizzle oil slowly into nut mixture while processing until the nut mixture becomes spreadable. Adding more oil will make the nut butter creamier.

Refrigerate and use to spread on crackers, apple slices, or for a nutritious breakfast on healthy toast. Keeps well if refrigerated.

Jane's Wheat-free Oatmeal Chip Cookies:

1 1/3 Cups oat flour

½ Tsp. salt

½ Tsp. baking soda

1 Cup buttery sticks (olive oil based spread)

1 Cup brown sugar

¼ Cup granulated sugar

1 egg

1 tsp. vanilla

¼ Cup water

1 Cup chopped walnuts

½ Cup raisins or dried cranberries

1 Cup carob chips

3 Cups rolled oats

Heat oven to 350 degrees. Sift flour, salt, and baking soda together. Beat butter, sugars, eggs, vanilla and water together until fluffy. Fold in flour mixture, add nuts, raisins, oats (one cup at a time). Drop by rounded teaspoons about two inches apart on a lightly greased cookie sheet. Bake twelve-fifteen minutes. Transfer to wire racks and cool. Makes about four dozen cookies. These freeze well and make a high fiber, valuable-fat, occasional treat. Spread a little almond butter on these cookies for an even more beneficial snack.

22. Listen Up! Bonus CD

To download your free CD, go to
http://www.riverlightcenter.com/freecd

Your password is: Winatlosing

Listen at least once a day while relaxing in a quiet place where you will be undisturbed. Never listen while driving or operating machinery!

Jane H. Percy, B.A., CIH, CHt, Neuro Trainer

Jane H. Percy is a certified hypnotherapist in private practice. Jane specializes in medical hypnosis, guided imagery, empowerment coaching, and past-life regression therapy She was a student of Dr. Brian Weiss. Jane is also a Certified Intuitive Healer. She 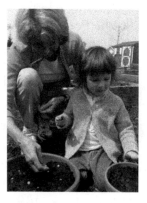 is a neuro trainer and director of Riverlight Brain Training Center in Stonington, CT.

Her work has been the subject of newspaper feature articles, an NBC TV broadcast, and several radio broadcasts. A writer, teacher, and noted guest speaker, Jane has created programs and seminars for Pfizer, The Alzheimer's Association, Child and Family Services, Backus Hospital, Hospice of Southeastern Connecticut, and the Lawrence And Memorial Hospital Wellness Center.

Prior to launching River Light Wellness Center, Jane was the founding director of the London Academy of Theater. During her six years as head of the conservatory acting and design program, which is now housed at Shakespeare's Globe Theater, Percy taught courses in presentation.

Jane's other theater credentials include stints as Director of International Programs at the Eugene O'Neill Theater Center, Waterford, Connecticut, where she created the first ever bi-lateral Eastern European theater projects in St. Petersburg, East Berlin, Warsaw, and Prague. Percy was also the Founding Director of The Moscow Semester.

Jane was Associate Director of Admission at Smith College, where she chaired the International Student Committee and served as advisor during the development of a dual degree engineering program for women.

Jane holds a BA in Music from Connecticut College and certification in Russian language from Dartmouth College. She is a Past Life Regression Therapist certified by Dr. Brian Weiss, an Intuitive Energy Healer certified by the Stillpoint Institute, and has National Guild of Hypnotists pain management, trauma and hypno-oncology certification. Jane has taught *Lighten Up! Win At Losing* classes at the William H. Backus Hospital, L&M Hospital Wellness Center and Riverlight Wellness Center. Jane is an avid sailor, gardener, painter and writer. She is the mother of two grown sons and has a granddaughter who loves healthy food!

BUY A SHARE OF THE FUTURE IN YOUR COMMUNITY

These certificates make great holiday, graduation and birthday gifts that can be personalized with the recipient's name. The cost of one S.H.A.R.E. or one square foot is $54.17. The personalized certificate is suitable for framing and will state the number of shares purchased and the amount of each share, as well as the recipient's name. The home that you participate in "building" will last for many years and will continue to grow in value.

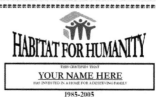

Here is a sample SHARE certificate:

HABITAT FOR HUMANITY

THIS CERTIFIES THAT
YOUR NAME HERE
HAS INVESTED IN A HOME FOR A DESERVING FAMILY

1985-2005

TWENTY YEARS OF BUILDING FUTURES IN OUR
COMMUNITY ONE HOME AT A TIME

1200 SQUARE FOOT HOUSE @ $65,000 = $54.17 PER SQUARE FOOT
This certificate represents a tax deductible donation. It has no cash value.

YES, I WOULD LIKE TO HELP!

*I support the work that Habitat for Humanity does and I want to be part of the excitement! As a donor, I will receive periodic updates on your construction activities but, more importantly, I know my gift will help a family in our community realize the dream of homeownership. **I would like to SHARE in your efforts against substandard housing in my community!** (Please print below)*

PLEASE SEND ME _____ SHARES at $54.17 EACH = $ $_____

In Honor Of: _____

Occasion: (Circle One)   HOLIDAY   BIRTHDAY   ANNIVERSARY

        OTHER: _____

Address of Recipient: _____

Gift From: _____ *Donor Address:* _____

Donor Email: _____

I AM ENCLOSING A CHECK FOR $ $_____ PAYABLE TO HABITAT FOR HUMANITY <u>OR</u> PLEASE CHARGE MY VISA OR MASTERCARD *(CIRCLE ONE)*

Card Number _____ Expiration Date: _____

Name as it appears on Credit Card _____ Charge Amount $ _____

Signature _____

Billing Address _____

Telephone # Day _____ Eve _____

PLEASE NOTE: Your contribution is tax-deductible to the fullest extent allowed by law.
Habitat for Humanity • P.O. Box 1443 • Newport News, VA 23601 • 757-596-5553
www.HelpHabitatforHumanity.org

CPSIA information can be obtained
at www.ICGtesting.com
Printed in the USA
JSHW081356190523
41962JS00001B/76